The Evolution of Essential Oils

Preventative Ways to Health

Dr. Marcy Foley

Published by:
INDIGO MEDIA
Provo, Utah
2005

ISBN
0-9762879-1-9

Editor: Markho Victor Rafael
Layout & Typesetting: skribble design

Printed and bound in the United States of America

Embracing Health
Using Plant Life Concentrates

You are about to embark upon the most exciting health discovery journey of your life! The purpose of this booklet is to teach you how to utilize the most *bio-available* form of herbal essences to assist you in attaining and maintaining your health goals. *Bio-available* means the most absorbable and utilizable form of a product to sustain our Life Force and our health.

We have used herbs as long as life has existed upon this planet. In the earlier times, when we were more in tune with nature, we would use herbs, florals (flowers), the barks and roots of trees, bushes, seeds and more, to bring us into a more complete connection to the Source which created us. As long as we have had records of the various civilizations on this planet, we note that herbs and spices have always been used to flavor their foods and beverages. They used these pure members of the plant kingdom for their healing, and also simply enjoyed their vibrational frequency to enhance their love and joy for living.

God gave us the herbal kingdom as a tool *(and beautiful gift)* for the purpose of reconnecting to our Source. Herbs are pure, innocent, and have a vital life force. When we disconnect from our higher frequency energies, we manifest disease within our bodies, as well as on our planet - our Earthly home. When we choose to connect with the herbal or nature kingdom, we have a direct tool to assist us in regaining our Life Force.

In order to accomplish this task, we must use herbs in their wholeness; herbs which are grown, prepared and delivered into our human bodies in their most natural state. The herbs must first be grown in soil which is rich in its natural properties. This means the herbs are not grown with the use of unnatural substances such as pesticides and chemical fertilizers. We need to use botanical materials that are prepared in a way which delivers all their essential nutrients.

My first health mentor, Rev. Hanna Kroeger, taught, "Herbs heal the *Spirit* of the body, which then filter down into our physical selves." She said that herbs, flowers, roots, the barks of trees, seeds and flowers get us in tune with our Creator, as long as the substances are pure, and not adulterated with various unhealthy ways of harvesting, processing and preserving them.

When a properly produced plant material is taken into the physical body, there is a corresponding *spiritually vitalizing* effect. This is the vibration which truly heals us! I believe we, as members of the human race, have as our purpose to understand and put into practice that which is our true nature - **Love**. As a demonstration of our appreciation and gratitude to our Creator, I also believe it is our duty to take care of our physical body and our health.

Love is the *God glue*, which unites us as the human race. When we get out of touch with the Plant Kingdom and with the Earth, we begin to lose our sense of the connectedness to Life. We lose our purpose for living this life and we don't feel like giving or contributing to our world, or even our family. We end up as sad, depressed, resentful, fearful and miserable human beings. We are sick in our body, heart, mind and spirit. This is why we have so many people on prescription drugs for insomnia, anxiety, depression, headaches, stress and a host of other maladies.

The plant kingdom is here to serve us (*or rescue us*), as humans, upon the Earth. It is as if these beautiful plant materials share their healing, loving attributes and gifts with humanity to help bring us back into balance. The key to healing any condition is to get back in balance - *The Law of Homeostasis*. I believe the use of the aqueous Plant Life Concentrates (hereafter referred to in this document as PLC's) is the easiest and most pleasurable way to maintain homeostasis.

In addition to using these precious gifts from the Plant Kingdom, we must also eat a natural, organic diet of fresh wholesome foods. God did not mean for us to process all the life force and nourishment out of the raw materials given to us for our physical sustenance. Excessive food processing is one of humanities greatest health disasters, which has given us fast foods and foods produced by factories that we simply re-heat in a microwave oven.

Many of us wonder why we are sick, and yet most of the "civilized" countries ingest, on a daily basis, refined sugars, refined and altered oils and trans fatty acids. We ingest grains that have the fiber, vitamins and minerals removed from them. We ingest fruit drinks that have added sugar, artificial flavors and preservatives. Many busy people succumb to using vegetables that are either canned or frozen, for our convenience. We are told to just boil them or put them in the microwave.

I find this terribly sad and boring! No wonder we eat so much? Our food has no flavor and little to no nutritional value. So we crave more food because we are unsatisfied and our body feels, in its intelligence, that if we eat more, we will certainly gain more nutritional value. However, most of us load up on nutrient-poor foods... and we feel more and more depressed, lethargic and uninterested in life.

Law of Signatures

The Plant Kingdom has a vital life force within it, because it is one of God's creations. I believe our Creator gave us plants to assist us in keeping our vibrational frequency at its highest potential in order to maintain our health and well-being.

Each plant species has a personality, just as we humans have a personality. This is called *The Law of Signatures - The Law of Signs*. Many of us may wonder how the ancient people knew what herb or flower to use for various conditions. God provided the Law of Signatures, so we could easily see the similarities between the plant kingdom and the human body.

To put into use the Law of Signatures, we look at the shape of the plant material, the color, the scent, and all aspects of this substance to direct us as to its use. The flower called bleeding heart, with its beautiful heart-shaped flowers, can help heal emotional heart wounds. Walnuts resemble the brain with its two "hemispheres" complete with a membrane (*similar to corpus callosum*) dividing the two halves, encased in a hard shell (*similar to the human skull*). Fruits and vegetables, which are red, have been shown to provide healing aspects to our blood and circulatory system. These include beets, tomatoes, and red grapes. There are countless other examples.

There are many ways plant materials can be made into substances we can ingest internally or use on the exterior of the body. Let's explore some of the ways we have utilized herbs, flowers, roots, bark, seeds, and resins. I will hereafter refer to these as "plant materials", which encompass all of these substances.

Preserving Plant Material
by Drying or Dehydrating

The most common way of preserving herbs has been to pick them from the garden, and then hang them upside down to dry. In large-scale operations of many herbal companies, the herbs are dehydrated (using heat) and then ground into a powder. I toured one well-known company with a very large facility. They actually had a whole room for each herb, into which they would blow the dried plant material for storage. Then, that material was transported to the place where it was put into capsules and packaged into bottles, to be sold to its distribution network.

I felt so sad when I saw this because there was no feeling of life, or of treating these beautiful herbs with reverence or love. When an herb is dried and put into capsules, the majority (from 85-95%) of the essential oil component is lost. I look at the essential oil as the highest life force within the herb, and that part which directs the entire plant substance as to how to act in the body.

When the essential oil is missing, we are just taking the dried herbal powder into the body. The body does not know as well how to make use of this substance. Sometimes people will take from 10 to 100 capsules of these herbs daily, thinking they are healing the body. In actuality, each of those capsules has to be made into a water-soluble form (like a tea) in the body for that substance to have the potential for it to work. Many times, a person actually makes matters worse by ingesting this many dried herbs in capsules because most of us are dehydrated to begin with. When this much dried plant material is taken into the body, it enhances the dehydration, and a healing crisis is the result! We are constipated and feel lethargic.

Water Extractions, Infusions and Decoctions

In this form of extraction, dried or fresh herbs are made into a tea. The herbs are put in a tea strainer or tea ball, and boiling water is poured over them. Commercial preparations use a tea bag, which you dunk in boiling water. When you make coffee, you grind the beans and pour boiling or hot water on top of the coffee grounds. These are either called water extractions or infusions. A decoction is made from tree bark, roots or seeds. They are boiled in a pan for 20 minutes, and up to several hours, before being strained for use.

Alcohol Extraction

Another way to extract the essences of the plant material is through the use of alcohol. Generally a wood or grain alcohol is used. Sometimes pure vodka or brandy is used. The resulting product is called a tincture. Some feel that this process pulls out more of certain properties within the plant material, that a water extraction cannot reach. The problem is that if we ingest too much of this type of extraction, the liver will have to detoxify the alcohol, which may cause adverse effects or nullify many of the health-promoting qualities from the tincture. Some people are also allergic to alcohol or don't wish to have any alcohol in their bodies.

Other Extractions

Instead of using alcohol, one can use glycerin, vinegar or an oil to extract the plant material. While these are not as toxic as using alcohol, these preparations still do not render all the properties in the plant material.

Chemical Extraction

Toxic chemicals are sometimes used to extract the plant material. The most common of which is hexane. This is a harsh technique, and while some claim that they can remove the hexane after the extraction has taken place, I don't believe all of it can be removed. I feel the energy of shock that takes place within the plant material when toxic chemicals are used will also stay within the extraction, and go into our bodies. We choose to ingest these lovely herbs and other plant materials for their high vibration and to take that gentle, powerful purity into our bodies. This type of extraction is a poor choice on many levels - not good for our body on a spiritual, physical, emotional or mental level. Using toxic chemicals to create health-promoting substances is also not a loving practice to the plant, and causes environmental damage to the Earth.

Poultices

A poultice is made when the plant material is ground up with the use of a mortar and pestle, and then mixed with a carrier substance. Common carrier substances include bee's wax, olive oil, glycerin, aloe Vera gel or lanolin. This type of preparation was created to get as much as possible of the plant material into the carrier substance, for the purpose of applying externally to the body for insect bites, tumors, painful joints, or for cosmetic usage.

Compresses

To make a compress the plant material is ground up with the use of a mortar and pestle. Or, in the case of aloe vera or comfrey, the leaves are bruised, and placed either directly on the skin, or placed between pieces of cheesecloth. Then a hot, wet cloth is placed over the compress, followed by a dry towel to keep the moisture in.

Distillation

For thousands of years, distillation has been used to produce the essential oil out of various plant materials. In this case a large distiller is employed. The dried plant material is put on top of a rack that sits above the boiling water. The material is cooked, under pressure, until the steam rises up to reach the condensing coils.

The liquid material is collected in a vat below the condensing coils. There are two substances collected - the floral water or hydrolet is the majority of the liquid, and on top of this floats the essential oils. They are called essential "oils" because they are lighter in molecular weight, and thus float on top of the hydrolet. Historically, the essential oils were considered the most important part, and often the hydrolet was thrown away, or used in external preparations as cosmetics or body care products. Only in recent times, have there been practitioners who are using these floral waters/hydrolets for various methods of healing.

I have been working with therapeutic quality essential oils nearly 10 years. I wrote a book entitled *Embraced by the Essence*, to describe how to use essential oils. I honestly did not ever believe I would find anything, which could ever compare with the power of essential oils. These are indeed wondrous substances that I truly love. At the same time, it is important to recognize that essential oils are a processed product. In the school of Natural Healing, I learned through Dr. John R. Christopher's teachings that we are to use herbs in their wholeness. Essential oils do not fit this definition.

Supercritical Fluid - CO_2 - Extraction

Now we have a totally new form of extraction. It uses harmless carbon dioxide gas, along with pressure., The gas reaches a supercritical fluid state and acts as a natural solvent. The oils and resins (oleoresins) are extracted from the herbs, the pressure is lowered and the supercritical fluid returns to CO_2 gas and is then reusable. It is a very clean, healthy and environmentally friendly process.

One important point of this type of extraction is that heat and chemical solvents are not necessary to create these extractions. In this way, the many health-promoting properties and the high frequency vibration inherent within the plant material are still intact with a vibrant life force!

Once the pure herbal oleoresins are captured, they are rendered water-soluble through a proprietary chemical-free emulsion technology. The process creates a concentrated, water-soluble essence from the whole plant that has maximum flavor and nutritional value and does not need refrigeration.

Since water is the delivery system, these whole plant essences can be added to pure water or anything else that could be improved by its flavors and nutritional value. Since our body is 60% - 70% water, and our brain is over 90% water, there could not be a better delivery system to the body than these aqueous Plant Life Concentrates (PLC's).

Comparison of the Old vs. New Paradigm in Processing Plant Materials

In the old paradigm ground herbs and spices had a limited shelf life. They were subject to the loss of volatile substances during dehydration and grinding. They were subject to further degradation and/or microbial growth over time. They lacked consistency, flavor and therapeutic properties within the plant material. They required heating or sautéing.

In the new paradigm, these aqueous PLC's have a very long shelf life. Unlike dried or ground spices and herbs the flavors will not evaporate over time. There is a consistency of flavor and the natural phyto-nutrients and therapeutic compounds remain intact. They are ready for instant use without heating or sautéing.

The Power of Aqueous Preparations of Oleoresins

I was privileged to have a powerful taste test of the oleoresin produced by the CO_2 extraction and compared that to the oleoresin made water-soluble. WOW! What a difference! I took a little dab on the end of my finger of the chili oleoresin and touched it to my tongue. It was hot, yet not dramatically so. And then I was given just a tiny dot (how much would adhere on the end of a toothpick) of chili, made into the aqueous substance, much smaller than my previous sample. It was dramatically more potent and caused a lot of heat on my tongue! Also, the aqueous substance was at least 10-20 times more diluted than the oleoresin.

Why was the more diluted form stronger in its flavor? *Because it was rendered water-soluble!* This means it was more available to all of the cells and fluids of my body, so my body was able to recognize and make use of what it was given! It does little use to ingest a material into the body, if the body can't make use of it.

Several years ago I heard a quote that Salt Lake City regularly has to remove at least two 55-gallon barrels of pills, tablets and capsules which have to be filtered out of their water processing stations. This comes from what we flush down the toilet! That means, these were supplements people paid good money for, and yet their bodies were unable to utilize. So, the body excreted them.

If we wish to operate within the optimum level of our health, we must ingest substances that our bodies can recognize, absorb and utilize. These aqueous Plant Life Concentrates are our ticket to health, vitality and well-being.

Food as Medicine

The famous doctor, Hippocrates, nearing the end of his long life in medicine declared, *"Let food be your medicine, let medicine be your food."* Because these substances are pure organic food products, the therapeutic value of ingesting the entire range of substances within the plant material can be fully available to everyone without government regulation.

Alive & Vibrant!

These Plant Life Concentrates (PLC's) are alive and vibrantly here to assist us in raising the frequency of our body. Some people who are able to tap into the energy of these substances can feel the life force within these substances without even opening the bottle! Healing takes place when we raise the frequency above that of the disease level. We cannot achieve this with dried, dead plant material or herbs that have been extracted with chemical solvents and high heat. When a plant material is dried, then stored in jars for years before use, its vibrant life force is long gone. How can we expect this material to enhance the vibrational frequency in our bodies?

What is Frequency?

Frequency is a measurable rate of electrical energy that is constant between two points. All atoms in the universe have vibrational motion, or electrical frequency. Frequency is the number of oscillations per second, and is measured in Hertz. Dr. Royal Raymond Rife said that all diseases have low frequency. We can change our tendency toward lower or depressed frequency, and the negativism that accompanies it, by the application of aqueous (water-soluble) PLC's, which carry higher frequencies that uplift the energies in the body.

Chapter Two:
The Importance of Digestion

We usually hear the phrase, "We are what we eat." I have altered this to say, "We are the product of what we eat, what we assimilate, and what we eliminate." No matter how good our diet is, if we are unable to assimilate (or make use of it), it is of no use to us.

There are many parts of our body involved in digestion. We begin with the saliva in our mouth, containing starch-digesting enzymes. Food is then transported into our stomach where a combination of grinding (mechanical action) is combined with protein-digesting enzymes (proteases). Food is next emptied into the small intestine, where carbohydrate-digesting alkaline enzymes (amylases) are secreted. Fat-digesting enzymes (lipases) are also provided. Food is moved through the small intestine, and slowly absorbed through the lining of the intestines to go into the blood. The end product of digestion is what we expel in our bowel movement.

The Importance of the Liver

Let's diverge here into one of the most important internal organs in the body - the liver. Notice that the first 4 letters of the word liver are LIVE. In fact, we would not be alive were it not for the thousands of functions our liver provides for us. Here is a list of some of the most important functions of the liver.

- As a digestive organ, the liver metabolizes proteins, fats and carbohydrates.
- The liver creates bile, which is an emulsifier of fats. Bile is concentrated and stored in the gall bladder
- The liver stores blood and energy reserves in the form of glycogen.
- The liver stores fat-soluble vitamins.
- The liver helps maintain electrolyte and fluid balance.
- The liver breaks down excess hormones (the most important of which is estrogen).
- The liver stores certain unresolved emotions - mostly anger, rage and resentment - or bitterness (a shared function with the gall bladder).
- The liver is the major detoxification organ through its various enzyme systems - thus its role as a blood-purifier.
- The liver transforms fat-soluble toxins into water-soluble substances, which are more easily eliminated.

One of the most important considerations in healing the liver is in the type and quality of fats and oils we ingest. This is because the liver is the main place in the body where fats and oils are processed. In the not-too-distant past, we consumed a majority of saturated fats through tropical oils and animal fats. Due to an incorrect interpretation of research, or not telling the true information of fats and oils by certain special interest groups (*motivated by greed and profit*), saturated fats were labeled as "bad", while polyunsaturated fats became "the good guys". We were told that saturated fats contributed to cardiovascular disease.

We don't have the space in this booklet to go into this discussion.[1] The fact is that traditional societies who have eaten saturated fats for hundreds or thousands of years have little heart disease, diabetes, or many other diseases common in the "civilized" societies, as long as they adhere to their traditional diets. The problem with unsaturated fats is their high degree of instability, thus their ease in becoming oxidized or becoming rancid in our bodies. This leads to cancer, premature aging, excessive skin wrinkles and liver damage. (*Refer to information on Free Radicals described later*).

There are many symptoms our body gives us as its way of communicating that the liver needs help -- that the liver is congested, toxic and unable to do its job. The following are a few examples:

- Feeling tired after eating
- PMS, as well as excessive menstrual flow containing many clots of blood
- Headaches
- Allergies
- Chemical and Environmental Sensitivities
- Mood Swings, especially involving depression and anger
- Night Sweats - not the same as hot flashes
- Immune System dysfunction & Auto-immune Disorders
- Obesity
- Flatulence (Intestinal gas)
- Inability to handle fats without feeling nauseated, and belching
- Chronic Fatigue, dizziness, heart palpitations, rapid pulse

[1] Please consult the Weston Price Foundation web site for more information on the healthy fats and Dr. Price's research into traditional diets and Health–http://www.westonaprice.org

- Irritability, anxiety, frustration and inability to function harmoniously with those around you
- Lack of harmonious flow of vital energies in your body. One minute you are "bouncing off the walls", and the next minute you are depressed and lethargic, barely able to climb a flight of stairs

Excitement and Enthusiasm for Loving Your Liver!

Do these two lists stimulate an excitement within you to pay some loving attention to your liver? You will notice that while the Plant Life Concentrates (PLC's) described in this booklet work on all 12 systems in the body, the majority of their functions focus upon digestion, antioxidant activities, and the nutritional qualities these extracts provide. Many of these PLC's also focus upon the liver. While using these PLC's, it is also important to remember the principles of a good natural foods diet. While we will not focus upon diet and nutrition in this book, we will outline a few basic principles.

General Principles of Diet and Nutrition

- Eat food as close as possible to how it was created. It is better to eat an apple than to chug a glass of apple juice. We can overdo it when drinking fruit and vegetable juices, even if they are 100% organic. If we chug a whole glass of juice, we don't mix it with our saliva, and it can cause a spike in our blood sugar, just as if you ate a high sugar product.

- Dr. John R. Christopher taught us, "Drink your solids and chew your liquids." This means to chew solid food in our mouth until we mix it with the salivary amylase. Also, swish liquids (other than water) in our mouth.

- Choose the highest quality you can find in your meats, grains, nuts, seeds, fruits and vegetables. This means they are organic, "chemical-free", "pesticide-free", and food that has not been genetically modified. Read all labels, as this is your way to discover if a food has added sugar, salt, hydrogenated oils, canola or soybean oil, stabilizers, enhancers, preservatives, etc. Preferably buy food that doesn't have a label, but is just plain food! Then chop it up and gently cook it, with love, adding PLC's to your meals, in your own kitchen. It can be a form of family bonding (and teaching children) to engage the whole family in the preparation of meals.

- Choose fresh fruits and vegetables over canned or frozen.

- Prepare food using a conventional stove top and oven, or convection/toaster oven. A microwave oven denatures proteins, which the body cannot use. It is some of these denatured proteins, which are often stored in the body and give nourishment to the formation of tumors, as well as a congested lymphatic system!

- Eat REAL FOOD that you cook instead of pre-prepared entrees, frozen box mixes and canned foods. These foods are often LOADED with "extras" that are detrimental to your health.

- Use healthy fats and oils. I recommend olive oil, raw cultured butter (from grass-fed cows), coconut oil and palm kernel oil.

- Use herbs and spices that are alive and vibrant! It is important to stimulate the 5 different taste buds, which are receptors for the 5 major flavors in foods, herbs and spices.

The 5 Flavor Qualities in Foods, Herbs and Spices

In the United States, we are advised to follow the "food pyramid", and eat our required amounts of the milk group, meat group, fruits and vegetables group, and breads and cereals group. No mention is made about flavor qualities of sweet, bitter, sour, acrid or salty. We have 5 different types of taste buds on our tongue, which are receptors for these flavors.[A] I believe our Creator put these receptors there for a reason, and that reason had more to do than simply enjoying the flavor of our food.

- **Acrid/Pungent/Spicy** substances have an affinity for the lungs where they open up the bronchioles and provide enhanced circulation. They also support the digestive and urinary systems.

- **Bitter** substances have an affinity for the heart. They provide stimulant and protective actions for the liver and digestive systems.

- **Salty** substances balance life at the level of the cell - helping to move certain substances into cells, and others out of cells. Life happens at the level of the cell. Salty substances have an affinity for the kidneys to keep our electrolytes and fluids in proper balance and also nourish the nervous system.

- **Sour** substances have an affinity for the liver, to aid in detoxification and protection of the cells and enzyme systems in the liver. They help balance pH, balance nerve cell communications and stimulate the activity of digestive enzymes.

- **Sweet** substances have an affinity for the spleen to support our immune system. They nourish cells and provide tone to the blood and digestive system.

[A] See Appendix A, Map of Taste Receptors Diagram

To provide optimum nourishment and stimulation to our entire body, it is important to have all of these tastes and properties present daily, if not all 5 in each meal.

In the Caucasian population of the USA, most of our foods are pretty bland and tasteless. Because our digestive systems are in such need of bitter substances, to help the liver, we ingest coffee. This is a bitter herb, and various coffees around the world have specific areas of the body they stimulate and nourish. The key is to ingest a small amount, just as with any other herb, and not over-do it. The addition of sugar and cream to this bitter herb defeats the purpose of the use of coffee as a therapeutic substance!

The Hispanic and Asian populations use more chili, onions and garlic, which the immune and cardiovascular systems love. The Black population in the South uses more greens, which the liver loves. The Asian and Indian populations use more of the bitter, sour and pungent spices of turmeric, cumin, cinnamon, cardamom and ginger. The Mediterranean populations use more of the green herbs, such as sage, rosemary, basil, thyme and oregano.

Most traditional (ethnic) cultures serve a portion of each of these substances within each meal. These come in the form of little dishes of pickles, sauces, fermented foods, various condiments, herbs and spices. Indian restaurants often have little bowls of cardamom and anise seeds, that one may chew after a meal to enhance digestion and freshen the breath.

When we stimulate the taste buds on our tongue with these 5 flavor qualities within our foods, herbs and spices, it sends a corresponding signal to the above-mentioned organs in the body. Thus, when we increase our use of certain aqueous PLC's, we favorably affect not only our taste buds; we more importantly stimulate the various digestive and other life-enhancing functions in our bodies.

Now, let us explore some of these PLC's, Culinary Herbs and substances that I believe will prevent major illnesses when used on a frequent basis. Remember, it is much easier to take care of us now, on a preventative level, rather than to abuse ourselves and hope to one day regain our health. Prevention is the place of power in healing!

Chapter Three:
Properties of Plant Life Concentrates

The following are the aqueous PLC's in this book and the Body Parts/Systems they nourish, stimulate and refresh.

PLANT	BRAIN NERVES	CARDIO-VASCULAR	DEGEN RESTORE	DETOX-ELIMIN	DIGEST-NUTRITION	EENT	EMOTIONAL
Allspice	X	X	X		X		
Astaxanthin	X	X	X	X			
Basil	X		X	X	X		
Cardamom	X				X		
Chamomile	X				X		
Chili	X	X	X				
Cinnamon	X	X		X	X	X	
Clove	X				X		
Frankincense		X	X		X		X
Garlic	X	X	X	X			
Geranium				X	X		X
Ginger	X		X	X	X	X	X
Green Tea		X					
Lemon	X		X	X			
Lemongrass		X			X		X
Lime							
Neroli	X				X		X
Nutmeg		X	X		X		
Onion	X	X	X				
Orange	X	X		X	X		X
Oregano	X						
Parsley	X				X		
Peppermint	X	X			X		
Rose	X	X					X
Sage	X	X	X				
Spearmint	X	X			X		
Thyme	X		X		X		
Turmeric	X	X	X	X	X	X	
Ylang Ylang		X					X

PLANT	ENDOCRINE	IMMUNE	MUSCLE BONES	REPRODUCTIVE	RESPIRA-	SKIN	URINARY
Allspice			X				
Astaxanthin	X	X					
Basil	X	X					
Cardamom		X					X
Chamomile			X	X		X	
Chili			X		X		
Cinnamon	X	X					X
Clove		X	X		X		
Frankincense	X	X			X	X	
Garlic		X			X		
Geranium	X	X					X
Ginger		X		X			
Green Tea	X	X	X				
Lemon		X	X		X		X
Lemongrass		X	X		X	X	X
Lime		X	X				
Neroli		X					
Nutmeg	X	X	X				
Onion	X	X					
Orange							X
Oregano		X	X		X		
Parsley				X			X
Peppermint		X			X		
Rose		X			X	X	
Sage		X			X		
Spearmint		X			X		
Thyme		X	X		X		
Turmeric	X	X	X				
Ylang Ylang	X				X		

What Are Free Radicals?

Before we begin our discussion of the individual plant materials, it is important to have an understanding about free radicals and antioxidants.[B]

The most deadly substance in our bodies is not a virus. It is a highly reactive molecule or molecular fragment called a free radical. Free Radicals are seeking areas of oxygen to complete their molecular structure. Thus, they occur when oxygen is oxidized (or burned) in the body. Free radicals travel trough cells, disrupting the structure of other molecules, causing cellular damage. Free radicals are molecules that are highly reactive to cells. Free radicals attack the cells of the body and the cell walls. They damage proteins, fats and nucleic acids in the body (RNA & DNA).

The liver has two enzyme systems (*Superoxide dismutase* (SOD) and *glutathione peroxidase*) in order to neutralize free radicals. However, since most of us have a damaged or compromised liver, it can't do its job properly. Thus, the rampant activity of free radicals causes the acceleration of the aging process. It is also logical to assume that if we have a high level of free radical activity in the body, which has damaged our genetic blueprint (DNA), we are more susceptible to cancer and many other degenerative disorders within the body.[2]

The signs of aging (and thus degeneration of the body) include loss of flexibility and normal joint motion - many "itis" diseases[3], hardening of the arteries, an opaque film developing over the eye (cataracts), degeneration of our protective enzyme systems in the liver, muscular and joint pain, chronic fatigue, allergies, chemical sensitivity, skin wrinkles, dry and cracked skin, lack of proper immune response, or auto-immune system disorders, sleep disorders, anxiety attacks, and much more.

[B] See Appendix B, Free Radicals Diagram

[2] I classify a degenerative condition as that which affects more than 2-3 body systems, and is a chronic, slowly evolving condition.

[3] Refer to Glossary. I use this phrase in reference to inflammatory conditions.

Free radicals occur in the body mostly due to our ingestion of oxidized fats and oils. This is due to our excessive intake of poly-unsaturated oils, eating fried foods and the intake of trans fatty acids. Also, free radical damage occurs due to excessive exercise, especially in highly polluted environments. Have you ever noticed that certain athletes, even though they are at or below their normal weight, tend to look much older than their age? Free radicals also come to us from exposure to pollutants in the air, preservatives, artificial fertilizers, processed foods, growth hormones in our meat, genetically modified foods, and also in our lack of eating enough fresh, raw food, fresh unadulterated herbs and spices.

What Are Antioxidants?

The solution to inhibiting free radical activity in the body is to ensure the highest levels of antioxidants in our diet, and minimizing the lifestyle activities that create free radical exposure. Antioxidants protect the cells and other bodily components by neutralizing the effects of free radicals. Antioxidants occur abundantly in the Nature/Botanical Kingdom in our fruits, vegetables and botanicals. *Please note the abundant antioxidants in the PLC's described shortly.*

The Systems and Categories of the Body

Rather than looking to simply alleviate symptoms of disease, I find it useful to see what systems of the body are affected in various healing challenges. In fact, we cannot really divide the body into categories and systems. The human body works as a whole, integrated unit. Each system interacts with each other.

The body systems are interdependent upon each other. So, as we work on one system, the other systems are benefited as well. The endocrine (hormonal) system controls the organ system.

The brain controls the endocrine, digestive, cardiovascular, respiratory and nervous systems. The nervous systems exert their controls over the muscular system and oversee the entire communication system in the body. There are feedback loops from the endocrine glands that communicate back to the brain, to redirect control mechanisms to the organs and glands, and on and on.

In recognizing the body, as a whole, I find it useful to look at the parts, which may be contributing factors in many disorders in the body. When dis-ease occurs, there are generally certain particular systems involved more than others. Therefore, I have divided the body into systems and categories as a study model. For instance, in wanting to heal arthritis, it may be useful to employ substances that help detoxify and rebuild the musculoskeletal and immune systems. Also, certain principles within degenerative conditions may also apply, such as balancing the pH, providing sufficient antioxidants, and other matters relating to the terrain theory of the body.

For the purposes of this booklet, I have created the following categories. Please note that in some cases a particular organ may exhibit many properties. For instance, the liver is part of the detoxification, immune and digestive systems.

- **Brain & Nervous System** - brain, autonomic, central and peripheral nervous systems

- **Cardiovascular System** - red blood cells, blood vessels (arteries & veins), heart

- **Degenerative/Restorative**

- **Detoxification & Elimination** - liver, colon

- **Digestive/Nutrition** - salivary glands, esophagus, stomach, liver, gall bladder, pancreas, small intestine

- **EENT** - ears, eyes, mouth, nose, sinus, teeth, throat

- **Emotional**

- **Endocrine System** - adrenals, ovaries, testes, pancreas, thymus, thyroid, pituitary, pineal

- **Immune System** - thymus, spleen, lymphatic system, tonsils, adenoids, white blood cells

- **Musculoskeletal System** - muscles, bones, connective tissues (tendons, ligaments), joints

- **Reproductive System** - ovaries, uterus, fallopian tubes, prostate, testicles

- **Respiratory System** - lungs, bronchi

- **Skin**

- **Urinary System** - kidneys, ureters, bladder

Glossary — Please refer to glossary at the end of booklet if you are unfamiliar with some of the terms used to describe the PLC's. The reason we have medical terminology is that it takes up less space, and uses fewer words to describe a condition. This is a small booklet, so I use these medical terms. I will list a couple of words here that I use often.

Pre-Glossary

- **Anti**—means "against", so if you see antibacterial, antiviral, antiparasitic, etc. it means this herb protects against bacteria, virus, and parasites - or if bacteria, virus or parasites are present, the herb can inactivate the "germ" or "bug".

- **Carminative**—a substance which causes intestinal gas (or flatulence) to be expelled

- **Expectorant**—causes you to cough up mucus

- **Flatulence**—intestinal gas

- **Mucolytic**—a substance that dissolves mucus

Combinations of Plant Life Concentrates

In the section which follows, I list some of the most important aqueous Plant Life Concentrates. In the ForeverGreen company, there are four different blends that I feel are excellent combinations of some of these PLC's. I will describe these first.

Green Dragon—green tea, chamomile, peppermint, spearmint, lemon, lemongrass, and parsley - This combination is useful in cleansing the blood, supporting the liver in detoxification and in alkalizing the body's pH. It is important to neutralize acidity within the body if we wish to be in optimum health. This combination is useful for oxygenating the cells and enhancing digestion.

Red Dragon—astaxanthin, ginger, orange, and sweet lime - This combination is a powerful antioxidant and can be supportive to the cardiovascular and immune systems. The PLC's in this mixture are supportive to brain, eye, heart and central nervous system (CNS).

White Dragon—cassia, cardamom, clove, lemon, nutmeg, allspice, ginger, and orange - This combination is antibacterial and antimicrobial. It assists the digestion, eases nausea, supports the immune system, and soothes stress and depression. It is strengthening to the intestinal system, enhances circulation and inflammatory processes. It can help to purify and detoxify the blood. It may also ease spasms and cramps.

Rainmaker—rose, neroli, ylang ylang and geranium - This combination is useful for emotional balance. Sipping on a mixture of this combination may provide useful support for those who live and work in stressful environments, as well as those who have a "sensitive" nervous system and feel a lot of internal anxiety.

Individual Plant Materials Described

Allspice—Contained in Red Dragon
Cardiovascular, Degenerative/Restorative, Digestive/ Nutrition, Musculoskeletal

Allspice takes its name from its aroma, reminiscent of a combination of spices - cinnamon, clove, ginger and nutmeg. It comes from an Evergreen tree, producing allspice berries, grown in the rainforests of South and Central America as well as in Jamaica. Allspice is high in *eugenol*, which is a strong antiseptic, antioxidant, and high in oxygenating compounds.

Astaxanthin—Contained in Red Dragon
Brain & Nervous System, Cardiovascular, Degenerative/Restorative, Endocrine, Immune, Musculoskeletal, Special Senses

Astaxanthin, with its strong red-orange pigment, is a naturally occurring carotenoid pigment found in aquatic life, which has strong antioxidant properties. It has antioxidant activity 10 times higher than beta-carotene and up to 1000 times higher than Vitamin E. Astaxanthin protects against oxidative damage of LDL-cholesterol, cellular and tissue membranes.

In the various underwater species where astaxanthin is found, research shows that astaxanthin exhibits a number of essential biological functions including protection against effects of UV light, protection against oxidation of essential polyunsaturated fatty acids, pro-vitamin A activity and vision, immune response as well as assistance in the reproductive cycles. We can only surmise that if it has these effects in the aquatic life forms, it might do similar things to the human population.

Astaxanthin has been shown to protect the retina from oxidative damage.[4] This could also include neuronal damage from retinal injury, or neuronal damage in age-related macular degeneration. As astaxanthin easily crosses the blood-brain barrier, it could also be useful in treating Alzheimer's, Parkinson's, spinal cord injuries and other types of central nervous system injuries.[5] There are numerous other benefits of astaxanthin.

Basil—*Brain & Nervous System, Immune, Digestive/Nutrition, Degenerative/Restorative, Detoxification & Elimination, Endocrine*

Basil herb is high in bioflavonoids and volatile (essential) oils. Flavonoids work at the cellular level to help protect chromosomes, cellular structures and also to protect against oxidative (free radical) damage. It is only when cholesterol and other fats are oxidized, that they cause damage in the body.

Basil has demonstrated strong antibacterial properties. One of basil's strongest components is eugenol, contained within the essential oil. Eugenol is a strong anti-inflammatory agent.

Cardamom—Contained in White Dragon
Brain & Nervous System, Digestive/Nutrition, Immune, Urinary

Cardamom is a member of the ginger family. It is more commonly used in the Middle East, India and China than in the United States. Cardamom is antiseptic, antiparasitic, antispasmodic, carminative, digestive, diuretic, and expectorant. It is also useful as a brain and nerve tonic.

Chamomile—Contained in Green Dragon
Brain & Nervous System, Digestive/Nutrition, Immune, Musculoskeletal, Reproductive, Skin

---

[4] Snodderly 1995

[5] Tso and Lamm 1996

33

This beautiful plant is cultivated in Germany, even though it is grown in many locations. Historically, chamomile has been a favorite and trusted remedy dating back to early Roman times. Chamomile is a mild herb mostly known for its soothing and calming properties. The flowering tops of chamomile are used to prepare a mild tea enjoyed as a mild sedative, and as a remedy for insomnia. It was used for skin conditions because of its anti-inflammatory properties, mostly from the essential oil component called *azulene*.

As a digestive aid, chamomile is a carminative. In Europe, chamomile is used in the form of bitters to stimulate ones appetite before meals. Chamomile is also used as an antispasmodic remedy for menstrual cramps. This herb is also helpful in liver detoxification and is mucolytic. Chamomile is a very safe herb, used in moderate amounts. If a person is allergic to asters, ragweed or chrysanthemums, they may have a sensitivity to chamomile products.

Chili—*Brain & Nervous System, Cardiovascular, Degenerative/ Restorative, Endocrine, Immune, Musculoskeletal, Respiratory*

Chili peppers go back as far as 7000 years of use in Central and South America. There are many types of chili peppers, with a very wide range in the hotness factor they produce. One of the most common myths about chili is that it causes stomach ulcers. In fact, the opposite is true. The main therapeutic substance in chili is called *capsaicin*, which provides the hotness factor and is capable of killing the bacteria H. Pylori, which is responsible for some types of stomach ulcers. Because of the heat present in chili, this is an excellent way to increase circulation as well as tissue respiration.

Capsaicin is also known for its anti-inflammatory and pain-reducing properties. It has been studied in the treatment for sensory nerve fiber disorders (such as diabetic neuropathy). By ingesting chili, you may help decrease your blood cholesterol levels, and prevent platelets from sticking together, causing the blood to thicken. We all know how well our sinuses work after eating a Mexican, Middle Eastern or Oriental meal in which chili is used. So, enjoy your chili peppers, and give your body a sensory thrill!

Cinnamon—*Brain & Nervous System, Cardiovascular, Detoxification & Elimination, Digestive/Nutrition, EENT, Endocrine, Immune, Urinary*

Cinnamon spice, made from the bark of the tree has several components that are responsible for its amazing healing and stimulating abilities. These include *cinnamic aldehyde, eugenol* (a member of the phenol group), and a few alcohol-based constituents. Cinnamon is a wonderful antioxidant. Cinnamon is strongly antiviral, antifungal and also antibacterial.

One of the most exciting aspects about cinnamon is in its ability to help Type II diabetics be less insulin-resistant by helping to free up the insulin receptor sites and only 1/2 teaspoon per day of cinnamon may do the trick.[6] This means it may not cure diabetes, but less insulin medication may be necessary, and blood sugar levels can be kept in better balance.[7]

Other studies show that cinnamon may be useful for the cardiovascular system by keeping blood platelets in a healthy condition. This means they only clump together when there is injury, not on an on-going basis, which can raise blood pressure due to blood that is too thick.

Within the GI tract cinnamon is a carminative, can help with urinary tract infections, and remove Candida albicans yeast overgrowth. It may help with menstrual pain and cramping. Cinnamon demonstrates anti-inflammatory activity, and also reduces triglyceride and LDL-cholesterol. Cinnamon may be taken internally in certain cases of fever, diarrhea or flatulence. Lastly, cinnamon has the ability to improve visual and cognitive motor skills, so it thus enhances the brain and nervous system.[8]

---

[6] *U.S. Agricultural Research Service*, December, 30, 2003.

[7] *Journal of Agricultural and Food Chemistry*, Anderson et al.

[8] Research discussed at the Association for Chemoreceptive Sciences by Dr. P. Zoladz, April, 2004.

Clove—Contained in White Dragon
Brain & Nervous System, Digestive/Nutrition, Immune,
Musculoskeletal

Clove bud has properties similar to cinnamon, and is also high in eugenol, which is its main chemical constituent. Many years ago in the United States, clove oil was used in the dental industry as an antiseptic and for pain control during dental surgery. It was used as an anti-inflammatory agent after tooth extraction or gum disease. Now a synthetic version is used. Like cinnamon, clove is an antioxidant, is antibacterial, antifungal and antiviral. It is a wonderful remedy for parasites, diarrhea, flatulence, and as an expectorant.

Frankincense—In Frankincense & Nutmeg blend
Brain & Nervous System, Cardiovascular, Degenerative/
Restorative, Digestive/Nutrition, Emotional, Endocrine,
Immune, Respiratory, Skin

Frankincense originated in the Middle East and has been used for thousands of years as an incense and religious ritual substance. The Biblical story is told about how frankincense, myrrh and gold were given to the Christ child. Frankincense is actually a resinous gum, which comes out of the frankincense tree. This was thought to be one of the earliest usages of the *Law of Signatures* noted. When the tree bark was cut, this substance oozed out of the tree to seal the wound, just as our blood clots to seal a skin wound.

Frankincense is very strong in its immunostimulant abilities, is antifungal, antibacterial and is also anti-infectious. It works as a tonic, wound healer and reduces fever. It has a strong reputation as having anti-tumor activities and the aqueous oleoresin can thus be rubbed externally on such areas of congested or congealed tissues. It also works on reducing external skin wrinkles.

For support of the musculoskeletal system, frankincense is anti-inflammatory and helps in many of the "itis" disorders. It is an astringent, (which increases nerve and muscle tone). Frankincense can help heal ulcerated tissue and is a well known expectorant and mucolytic.

Because the active ingredient in the aqueous oleoresin of frankincense crosses through the blood-brain barrier, frankincense works very well in the brain. It travels directly to the pineal and pituitary glands to help detoxify and rebuild these important areas in the brain. Thus, frankincense has been used to help alleviate depression and boost low energy levels in the brain and other areas of the body. Some report that when taking the aqueous oleoresin of frankincense, they feel more capable of giving and receiving love and notice an enhanced sense of well-being. As well as providing positive, uplifting energy, frankincense is also a mild sedative, to calm frayed nerves. Indeed, this substance is "more precious than gold," as it was said in the old days when frankincense was carried by camel caravans along the longest trade route in the world!

Garlic—*Cardiovascular, Degenerative/Restorative, Detoxification & Elimination, Immune, Respiratory*

Garlic has been called a natural antibiotic for hundreds of years to build up the immune system. It is antibacterial, and was used in great quantity in the days before refrigeration was available, to prevent food poisoning in many developing countries. Garlic has strong effects within the cardiovascular system. It regulates blood pressure, reduces clumping of platelets, reduces serum triglyceride levels and protect against oxidation of LDL-cholesterol.

Garlic protects two enzyme systems in the liver - *Glutathione Peroxidase* and *Glutatione-S-transferase*, which provide antioxidant functions. It also helps detoxify heavy metals in the system, inhibits prostaglandin formation (*because it is high in vitamin B6*) and lowers *homocysteine* levels which means it exhibits anti-inflammatory effects.

Geranium—Contained in Rainmaker Blend
Brain & Nervous System, Detoxification & Elimination, Digestive/Nutrition, Emotional, Endocrine, Immune, Skin, Urinary

Geranium is a common houseplant and is well known for its gentle properties on the skin and nervous system. It is antifungal and has astringent properties to draw together tissues that have become flaccid or have fatty deposits, which weaken the integrity of the tissue. Geranium dilates the bile ducts for the free flowing of bile, for the digestion of fats, and to help ease gallstones. Geranium also helps with liver detoxification, the reduction of jaundice and helps in other important liver processes. Geranium has been of help in Type II diabetes and for overall pancreatic support, as well as enhancement of the entire endocrine system.

Geranium has been called a great wound healer. On a physical level, it can stop bleeding from a wound. On an emotional and spiritual level, it can soothe the effects from traumatic experiences, and can leave the recipient with an overall sense of well-being and harmony. Geranium is refreshing and relaxing for the brain and nervous system.

Ginger—Contained in Red Dragon
Degenerative/Restorative, Detoxification & Elimination, EENT, Digestive/Nutrition, Emotional, Immune, Reproductive

Ginger is most commonly known for its action in the digestive tract where it soothes GI disorders, is a carminative, reduces intestinal spasms, is a strong antioxidant and anti-parasitic agent. Ginger has been found beneficial to reduce motion sickness, nausea, and cold sweats associated with anxiety and vomiting from a nervous stomach. It also helps relieve morning sickness in pregnancy.

Ginger contains anti-inflammatory compounds in its primary constituent called gingerol. Two studies demonstrated ginger helped reduce pain and swelling in those suffering from osteoarthritis and rheumatoid arthritis.[9] Ginger can also help reduce cramps during menstruation. It helps in detoxification and strengthening of liver tissue and can lower cholesterol levels. Ginger can also be useful as a mood enhancer.

Green Tea—Contained in Green Dragon
Brain & Nervous System, Cardiovascular, Endocrine, Immune, Musculoskeletal

Green tea is abundant in flavonoids, including polyphenolic catechins and other substances. These catechins are antibacterial, lower cholesterol, prevent heart disease and inhibit the enzymes involved in the production of free radicals in the inner arterial lining.[10] This lining (*called the endothelium*) is the thickness of only one-cell which delineates the space between the bloodstream and the wall of the artery where plaques can form. By protecting the endothelium from free radical damage, green tea catechins help prevent the development of cardiovascular disease. Though green tea contains caffeine, it is only about half that found in coffee.

Other cardiovascular properties of green tea include keeping the blood at the proper viscosity (degree of thickness) to help prevent blood clots. It can help lower blood pressure and help protect against kidney disease. Green tea helps protect the kidneys and liver from damage due to alcohol and other harmful chemicals. It also promotes fat loss.

Lemon—Contained in White Dragon
Cardiovascular, Degenerative/Restorative, Immune, Musculoskeletal, Respiratory, Skin, Urinary

---

[9] *Life Sciences,* December 2003; *Radiation Research,* January 28, 2004.

[10] *Biochemistry Biophs Res. Commun.* 2003 Oct 24: 3103:715-9

Lemon is a wonderful acid-neutralizer and has been used for both ulcerated tissue and heartburn. It is antibacterial, anti-infections, antiparasitic, and antiviral. It is a stimulant, and is warming to the body, helping to increase circulation. Lemon can remove excess fluids and mucus from the body. It helps in the formation of red blood cells, and can also stop bleeding if applied externally to a wound. Lemon is helpful in strengthening weakened vein walls (*thus helping varicose veins*) and can also enhance the quality of the skin. The liver loves the bitter qualities in lemon.

Lemongrass—*Brain & Nervous System, Immune, Degenerative/ Restorative, Detoxification & Elimination, Digestive/ Nutrition, Emotional, Respiratory*

While lemongrass smells like the lemon fruit, it is an herb that demonstrates antibacterial, antifungal and antispasmodic qualities. Lemongrass can help enhance lymphatic circulation, is mucolytic, and can thus support the immune system. It can relieve headaches, dispel nervousness and ease cramps. Lemongrass can help boost one's mood and is useful in treating depression.

Lime—Contained in Red Dragon
Immune, Musculoskeletal

Lime is antioxidant, antispasmodic and antiviral. Lime, similar to lemon, is also supportive to the liver.

Neroli—Contained in Rainmaker
Digestive/Nutrition, Emotional, Immune

Neroli comes from the beautiful flowers in the orange tree, before they form into an orange. Most of the actions of the florals are for emotional and spiritual balance. Neroli helps one to feel calm and tune into the love within. It can help replace depression, anxiety and nervousness with an overall sense of well-being, and that everything is going to favorably work out. On a physical level Neroli is also a digestive aid and is antibacterial, anti-infectious, antiparasitic and antiviral.

Nutmeg—In Frankincense & Nutmeg blend
Brain & Nervous System, Cardiovascular, Degenerative/ Regenerative Digestive/Nutrition, Endocrine, Immune, Musculoskeletal

One of the most important actions of nutmeg is the support it delivers to the adrenal glands. These tiny triangular-shaped glands sit above each kidney and produce hormones related to the "fight or flight" syndrome. This quality would be useful if one lived in the jungle and needed to run from a tiger. However, many of us live in this high anxiety state too often. Our adrenal glands are depleted, and then the body goes to the thyroid to try to pump out more energy, until the thyroid is depleted. Nutmeg can also help to nourish the nervous system, especially from chronic exhaustion and nervous fatigue.

Nutmeg is a digestive aid, especially for starches and fats. It can help to relieve nausea, diarrhea and vomiting. It is a carminative and can work to dispel gallstones. Nutmeg is antibacterial, anti-inflammatory and antiparasitic. It can help in cases of joint inflammation, can help ease muscular aches and pains and enhance circulation. Nutmeg also works quite well in supporting and nourishing the brain, along with Frankincense.

Onion—*Cardiovascular, Degenerative/Restorative, Endocrine, Immune, Respiratory*

Onion has similar qualities as Garlic. They are both sulfur-containing compounds. Sulfur has strong detoxifying and restorative effects, which is why people visit the various hot sulfur mineral springs to rejuvenate, and ease muscle and joint pains. Onion is antibacterial and anti-inflammatory. It inhibits prostaglandin activity, which accounts for the reduced pain and inflammation associated with the "itis" disorders.

Onion is high in the flavonoid called *quercitin*. Flavonoids (or bioflavonoids) enhance the body's ability to get Vitamin C into the cells. This constituent has the ability to dilate capillaries, so that the anti-inflammatory and antioxidant protective properties can be utilized. Flavonoids also help the cells to become more permeable, in order to get nutrients into cells and help toxins exit the cell. Quercitin has also shown the ability to stop tumor growth.

Onion is good for the immune and cardiovascular systems, and can lower high cholesterol levels. It helps normalize blood pressure in order to reduce the risk of arteriosclerosis, heart attack and stroke.

Onion also has many properties that help in diabetes, reducing the risk of diabetic heart disease, and also lower blood sugar levels. It does this by making the available insulin more able to assist the cells in regulating blood glucose levels. The fact that onion is high in the mineral chromium also adds to its blood sugar regulative abilities. In addition onion helps increase HDL-cholesterol while lowering cholesterol and triglyceride levels.

Orange—Contained in Red Dragon

Brain & Nervous System, Cardiovascular, Detoxification & Elimination, Digestive/Nutrition, Emotional, Immune, Urinary

Orange, as a member of the citrus family, is also high in flavonoids. It is antibacterial and an antioxidant. Orange helps increase circulation in the cardiovascular system, and can help reduce or prevent cardiac spasms and heart palpitations. Orange helps in the detoxification process. It can ease diarrhea, increase lymphatic circulation, thus regulating fluid and electrolyte levels in the body. It is also helpful for relieving fever, cold and flu symptoms, because it induces perspiration. Orange is useful when a woman is going through her menopausal experiences.

Remember, the orange fruit started out as the flower, from which we get the Neroli floral. So, on the emotional level, orange also helps bring joy, peace and tranquility to the heart in times of emotional distress. Orange has slight sedative qualities for easing anxiety.

Oregano—*Brain & Nervous System, Endocrine, Immune, Respiratory*

Oregano is high in numerous chemical constituents - thymol, carvacrol and rosminaric acid which contribute to its main actions on the immune system. It is a very strong antiviral agent and also exhibits antibacterial, antifungal and antioxidant properties. Oregano provides antiseptic qualities to the respiratory system. It can aid mental balance and enhance the metabolism of the body.

Parsley—Contained in Green Dragon
Brain & Nervous System, Digestive/Nutrition, Reproductive, Urinary

Parsley has a history of over 2000 years as a common garden herb, related to the carrot. One of its main functions is to alkalize the body. Its seeds are used as a carminative, and to enhance the digestive process. The root has been used as a diuretic and to regulate fluid and electrolyte balance. It can also help in urinary tract and kidney infections.

Parsley herb can also act as a mucolytic expectorant, thus reliving congestion in the respiratory tract. Because of its high chlorophyll content, it can help freshen the breath, because it cleanses the bloodstream. Parsley can also stimulate menstrual flow.

Peppermint—Contained in Green dragon
Brain & Nervous System, Cardiovascular, Digestive/Nutrition, Immune, Musculoskeletal, Respiratory

Peppermint is most well known for its actions in the digestive system for its carminative actions, heartburn relief, and its soothing qualities to the entire GI (gastrointestinal) tract. It can help in cases of nausea and vomiting. Peppermint is useful in diarrhea management. It can help in cases of irritable bowel syndrome.

Peppermint is antispasmodic, anti-inflammatory and antiseptic. It is an assistant to the liver for detoxification, and blood purifying properties. Peppermint is very useful for the respiratory system, to open up the bronchial tubes.

Peppermint helps alkalize the body, reduces fevers, and relieves headaches, especially migraines. It helps reduce hot flashes and creates menstrual regularity. Peppermint can stop internal and external bleeding.

Rose—Contained in Rainmaker
Cardiovascular, Emotional, Immune, Respiratory, Skin

Rose has the highest frequency of any floral extract. Its main actions center on emotional balance so that one often feels an increased sense of self-love and well-being. In addition, rose also is anti-infectious, helps stop bleeding, and is a brain stimulant. Rose can ease gingivitis and is wonderfully nourishing to the skin to ease or relax external skin wrinkles. It can also help in wound healing and for ulcer care.

Rosemary—*Brain & Nervous System, Cardiovascular, Digestive/ Nutrition, Immune, Reproductive, Respiratory*

Rosemary is most known for its ability to stimulate and refresh the brain. These qualities include an increased memory, enhanced mental sharpness, concentration and clarity. It can help decrease mental fatigue and stress. In addition, rosemary helps enhance circulation, and is used as a digestive aid. Rosemary helps relieve catarrh and mucus. It stimulates the immune system by being antibacterial, anti-infectious, antiviral, anti-inflammatory and antispasmodic. It has been used in France for ridding the body of excessive levels of Candida albicans (a yeast-fungus).

For the cardiovascular system, rosemary can help to regulate blood pressure. It can help to regulate the reproductive system through positive stimulation to the ovaries, for menstruation as well as testicular regulation. For the respiratory system, rosemary can help dispel excess mucus, and is also useful in working with sinusitis and bronchitis. It can also help reduce cellulite and help with fluid balance.

Sage—*Brain & Nervous System, Cardiovascular, Degenerative/ Restorative, Immune, Respiratory*

Sage is closely related to rosemary, and also has similar enhancements to the brain and nervous system. Sage enhances mental clarity and concentration while decreasing mental fatigue and depression.[11] Sage is soothing for the nervous and endocrine systems. Sage helps activate the adrenal cortex, and can help alleviate night sweats. It can help balance glandular functions related to estrogen, progesterone and testosterone. However, sage is stronger in its estrogen-like properties, so if one is estrogen-dominate, this herb needs to be used in moderate amounts. Sage can help in cases of menstrual irregularity and menopause.[12]

Sage is antibacterial and antiseptic. It also helps to reduce inflammatory responses and is an antioxidant. It also contains antioxidant enzymes, particularly *peroxidase* and *superoxide dismutase (SOD)*, which aid the liver. It contains flavonoids and enzymes related to oxygen usage. Therefore sage helps to stabilize the positive aspects of oxygen metabolism in the body, meanwhile disabling the negative aspects of oxidative damage within cells, leading to early aging. Sage can stimulate the metabolism. It has also been used to clear skin conditions such as eczema, acne, dandruff and hair loss.

---

[11] *Pharmacological Biochemical Behavior,* June 2003

[12] For more information on hormonal regulation, please consult Dr. Judi Gerstung's book

Spearmint—Contained in Green Dragon
*Brain & Nervous System, Cardiovascular, Digestive/
Nutrition, Endocrine, Immune, Musculoskeletal, Respiratory*

For the immune system, spearmint is antibacterial, anti-septic, antiparasitic, antispasmodic, and antifungal. It functions in the digestive system as a carminative, and to help alleviate nausea. It can help stop spasms - such a hiccough, and colic. Spearmint can enhance the respiratory system and also regulate blood pressure.

The endocrine system functions of spearmint are to regulate the hormones and speed up metabolic rate. On an emotional level, spearmint may help restore a sense of balance.

Thyme—*Brain & Nervous System, Degenerative/Restorative, Digestive/Nutrition, Immune, Musculoskeletal, Respiratory, Skin*

As an antibacterial agent, thyme can ease cases of bronchitis, coughs and chest congestion. Thyme is strongly antiviral, antifungal, antiparasitic, anti-inflammatory and antiseptic. For the brain and nervous system, it can help lessen nervous fatigue, stress, as well as general fatigue in the body. Thyme is especially useful after a long illness, when the body needs to regain its strength.
Thyme helps increase DHA levels in the brain, kidney and heart. As an antioxidant, it can help retard the aging process, as it also helps protect healthy fats in cellular metabolism.

Turmeric—*Brain & Nervous System, Cardiovascular, Degenerative/Restorative, Detoxification & Elimination, Digestive/Nutrition, EENT, Endocrine, Immune, Musculoskeletal*

Turmeric is a yellow root that has a long history of usage in India, Indonesia and China. The yellow-orange pigment in turmeric is called *curcumin*. This is an anti-inflammatory compound, which has research relating it to assisting in cases of irritable bowel syndrome, Chron's disease and ulcerative colitis. Curcumin helps lower *homocysteine* levels, which cause inflammation and irritation in the body. Turmeric is a powerful anti-oxidant to help protect cells and membranes, particularly helpful in the "itis" conditions. It can help ease joint swelling and morning stiffness.

Turmeric can help the liver detoxify *xenobiotic* (artificial estrogen-like) substances. This is of particular importance in today's estrogen-dominant society. Turmeric can help prevent the oxidation of cholesterol. It is when cholesterol, and other fats are oxidized, that they cause their damage to blood vessels. Turmeric can protect healthy fats in cell membranes, and is also anti-hemorrhagic. It helps protect DNA against damage.

Turmeric can also help protect against neurological disorders, including dementia, MS (*because it helps protect the myelin sheath*), Cystic Fibrosis, and Alzheimer's.[13] Curcumin protects against free-radical activity in the brain. Turmeric helps prevent plaque formation in the brain, leading to better communication within the brain.

In the respiratory system, turmeric is an ancient Ayurvedic herb to help with many conditions in the lungs and chest, decreasing congestion, coughs, chest pain and inflammation.

Ylang Ylang—Contained in Rainmaker
Brain & Nervous System, Emotional, Endocrine, Cardiovascular, Respiratory

---

[13] *Italian Journal of Biochemistry,* December 2003

Ylang Ylang is a beautiful flower, which works in the brain and nervous system to help ease depression, mental fatigue, is relaxing and can help with insomnia. It is used in emotional balancing, giving the recipient a feeling of safety and comfort.

It can help in Type II diabetes, tachycardia, heart palpitations and hypertension. Ylang Ylang is a balancer - of emotions, as well as cycles and rhythms in the body - blood pressure, acid/alkaline balance, breathing and also the yin and yang balance.

Chapter Four
Applications and How
to Use these PLC's

Now that we have explored the Plant Life Concentrates and their properties, let us see how we can benefit from their health-enhancing effects. My suggestion is to use these aqueous preparations in as many ways as possible, on an on-going basis, *according to your tolerance.* **Please remember that these substances (although foods) are very concentrated and potent.** If you have never used essential oils, or never worked much with strong herbal preparations, start slowly and build up. Here are a few ideas on how to get started enhancing your health and pleasure to your senses. *Please add your own!* I welcome you to e-mail me with ways you have found to use these substances, other than what I have provided here.[14]

Washing Produce and Meat to Reduce Bacteria

When you bring your vegetables home from the store or Farmer's Market, soak them in one of these PLC's: rosemary, sage, thyme. Even with organic chicken, I like to soak it in warm water mixed with rosemary or sage before cooking to reduce or remove bacteria.

---

[14] Please see my contact information at the end of this booklet.

Salad Dressings

There are endless possibilities of delicious salad dressings you can create using basil, chili, cinnamon, garlic, ginger, lemongrass, onion, rosemary, sage, thyme, and turmeric. I like to make my own mayonnaise using organic eggs and the type of oil and vinegar I choose. Most commercial mayonnaise has canola or soy oil, and sometimes a refined vinegar, which is acidic. I keep a jar of this homemade mayonnaise in the refrigerator. Then when I want to make salad dressing, I add 2 tablespoons walnut oil, 3-4 tablespoons organic balsamic or apple cider vinegar (both are alkalizing), one teaspoon homemade mayonnaise, and approximately 1/8th of a teaspoon each of garlic and basil. I make small batches of salad dressing that will only last 1-3 days, so I can use a different PLC the next time, or a combination of them! *I encourage you to "play" in the kitchen and see what you can create.*

Topical Applications

These PLC's can be used as one would use essential oils, by applying on location and massaging them in. Instead of using a vegetable oil, which would slow absorption of the PLC's, try using aloe vera juice or gel. Vegetable glycerin is another choice. When the area begins to get dry, spray with water, while you continue your massage. You can massage the back, feet, arms and legs in this manner. If you feel the area which was massaged is sticky, have recipient take a bath afterwards. This way you get to enjoy the extracts a little longer. Remember that certain plant materials can produce heat. Ginger is one of these. It will stay warm over the area for many hours. If you apply too much, when you get in the bath, it may increase the heat factor. If so, just keep gently dipping the area in the bath water, and the heat will soon dissipate.

Facial Mask - For Men and Women

In a small bowl place two teaspoons tsp dry clay. I like to use the French green clay. On top of this add _ tsp of the frankincense and nutmeg combination. Add sufficient water to make a paste that will adhere to the face and neck. You can apply with your fingers, or a little facial brush. Allow the mixture to stay on the face until it dries. Then fill the bathtub and put your face under the water to come off. Now you get to enjoy the clay and frankincense to vibrationally enhance your bath experience. If you don't wish to take a bath, you may simply wash the mask off in the sink. When out of the bath, be sure to put some moisturizer on your skin.

About the Cleansing, Detoxification and Refreshing Experiences

It is useful to realize that when you cleanse any part of the body, and abstain from your usual diet, you may experience emotions that come to the surface. These emotions have been stored in a cellular memory within the cells of the organ, and wish to be felt, acknowledged, honored, and loved. You may wish to record your experiences in a journal for further healing explorations.

I highly recommend, no matter what else you are doing during your refreshing cleansing experiences, that you use Rainmaker several times a day. These gentle florals of rose, neroli, ylang ylang and geranium are very supportive to any cleansing experience. As you cleanse on a physical level, you will concurrently cleanse on the emotional and spiritual levels as well. This is a wonderful opportunity to engage in prayer and meditation to talk to and listen to your Creator.

If you have never abstained from solid food, there could be some fear or anxiety present. While it is not true, you may *feel as if* you will "starve" or that you will be so uncomfortable you just can't tolerate this. Remember to work gently with your beautiful emotions. All emotional responses are real, however they may not always be true. What I mean by this is that if you experience an emotion, it is *real* for you. *Don't let anyone invalidate your emotional experiences.* Your job is to honor what comes up for you. At the same time, it is not true that you will actually starve by fasting a couple of days on these various juices and PLC's.

Most of the time, after a half day or so of doing your cleanse, or by the second day, you will really enjoy the experience. If you have never fasted before, choose one of the following cleansing refreshers that are only one day. Even if the cleanse suggests 1-3 days, you can gain benefit from doing it only one day.

Remember, obtaining and maintaining health is meant to be a fun and pleasurable experience! When you do these cleansing procedures for yourself, you will feel so good about yourself on an emotional and spiritual level. This will then filter down to your physical sense of wellness!

Herbal Compress for Decongestion

This procedure can be used over the intestines, kidneys, lungs, stiff joints, or anywhere in the body where there is congestion. Make a mixture or one teaspoon aqueous ginger oleoresin (PLC) to one quart very warm (not boiling) pure water. Don't use city water with contaminants. Soak a pure cotton cloth (*preferably all organic material*) in this ginger mixture. Cover area. On top of this place a warm towel which is moist, and cover with a dry cotton towel. If you have a hot water bottle, you can place this on top, to keep the mixture hot. Do this procedure for 30-60 minutes. In severe cases of congestion, this process can be done 2-3 times per day. In a preventative model, use this mixture once every 3-4 months. ***Note that this compress can use other PLC's such as Rosemary, Onion, Garlic, etc.***

Bathing as an On-Going Preventative Measure

One may use basil, oregano, rosemary, sage, thyme, (or a combination of each) in a bath. *I don't recommend using Chili, Ginger or Turmeric in the tub.* Use approximately one tablespoonful of the mixture of PLC's. Add to the bath water, and soak for 30-45 minutes. This process may be done as often as you desire. I suggest at least once every week.

Remember that as you soak in the tub, you will be exchanging fluids, having toxins exit and nutrients enter your body through the pores of your skin. It is important to continue hydrating yourself. Have a one-quart container of alkaline (8-9 pH) water to drink. Yes, you can also put any of the PLC's in your water, however if you are sensitive to too much stimulation, I suggest using the PLC's only in the tub and drinking plain water.

After this bath please go to bed and rest at least 30-60 minutes, or go directly to sleep. Place dry towels on the bed, as you will perspire. As you are relaxing, you focus on your wellness goals.

Foot Bath

As an alternative, for those who are unable to get in a bath tub, or don't have one available, you can do a foot bath. Get a large tub, as deep as possible, so you can have the most exposure to your skin. Fill with the hottest water you can tolerate, and add the PLC's to water. Soak 30-40 minutes, or until water becomes too cool.

Natural Sweetener - Yacon

To the various cleansing refreshers listed below, you may choose to add a sweetener. I suggest something which is natural, not refined, and measures the lowest on the glycemic index. Yacon is a root from Peru, and a relative of the sunflower plant. It is also a *prebiotic*, which means it is a food for the *probiotics* (the friendly intestinal flora). When one ingests a prebiotic, it helps the intestinal flora to reproduce, and thus stay at the optimal level within the intestines.

Yacon registers at approximately one (1) on the glycemic index. This means it has minimal (if any) effect of stimulating the release of insulin. Yacon has a pleasant taste, similar to molasses. Other good choices for a sweetener include Agave (or a mixture of Yacon & Agave), Stevia, Honey or Maple Syrup. The ForeverGreen company is the only source I have ever found Yacon. They also have a mixture of Yacon and Agave called Yakave.

Brain & Nervous System Refreshment

Mix together 1/2 teaspoon each of Basil, Rosemary, Sage, and 1/4 teaspoon of a mixture of Frankincense & Nutmeg. Use enough water for your volume of hair. For some it will be 2 tablespoons, for others it will be 1/2 cup of pure water. Apply to scalp. Massage in. Cover head with plastic shower cap, or a moist towel, followed by a dry towel on your shoulders. Leave on hair and scalp for 30-60 minutes. Then take a bath or shower and wash hair.

Cardiovascular & Circulatory System Refresher (Blood, Blood Vessels, Heart)

The blood is our river of life and vitality flowing to each of the cells, tissues and membranes of our body. If our blood is too thick, (because of platelet aggregation, heavy fats and cholesterol, triglycerides, and rampant with free radicals), we cannot be in good health. Therefore we need to keep our bloodstream as pure as possible. As you can see from the descriptions of the PLC's in the previous section, there are many possibilities to cleanse our bloodstream.

The following aqueous Plant Life Concentrates are supportive to the heart and circulatory system: chili, cinnamon, onion, garlic, green tea, turmeric, rosemary, ylang ylang, rose, Rainmaker, Green Dragon, Red Dragon. I suggest that once every other month we go on a one-day refresher program to cleanse our blood and open up our respiratory system.

This is a two part process — drinking the gallon of PLC-enhanced water *one day out of the month*, and the chest compress in the evening before you go to sleep.

Month One: Mix together one teaspoon of the White Dragon mixed with 1/2 teaspoon each of onion and garlic into a one-gallon container of pure water or apple juice/cider and the sweetener of your choice (or you can sweeten with grape juice). Make juice fresh if you have a juicer. Sip this mixture throughout the day. If you are hungry, eat raw apples, carrots, celery, radishes, green pepper, etc. Refrain from eating fats, grains or proteins.

Month Three: Mix together one teaspoon of the Green Dragon mixed with 1/2 teaspoon each of Cinnamon and Ginger. Mix in pure water, apple juice, carrot juice, or grape juice. If you are hungry, eat raw apples, carrots, celery, radishes, green pepper, etc. Refrain from eating fats, grains or proteins.

Month Six: Mix together one teaspoon each of the Red Dragon and the Emotional Blend mixture. Add 1/2 teaspoon chili (or 1/4 tsp chili and 1/4 tsp lemongrass) and mix into the water or juice of your choice - preferably a berry mixture (cranberry, raspberry, pomegranate). If you are hungry, eat raw organic grapes, strawberries, raspberries, blueberries or boysenberries, etc. Refrain from eating fats, grains or proteins.

PLC Compress: For each time you do the blood cleanse, do a different chest compress. I recommend Rosemary, Sage & Thyme, though you may make your own choices. Before going to bed, apply the PLC compress of your choice to the chest. Massage into the chest 1/8 to 1/4 tsp. of the PLC you are using. Then cover with a hot, moist cloth. When ready for bed, after the hot towel has cooled, remove towels and immediately go to sleep. The heat from the moist cloth helps to open the pores of the skin to allow the herb to more easily enter deeply into the tissue. It also provides some aromatic enjoyment, as the heat allows the beautiful vapors to reach your nose.

Detoxification & Elimination
Cleanse & Refresher
Enhances Entire GI Tract and Digestion

This is a 3-7 day program, depending on your level of determination, and your health condition. I recommend doing this once every 3 months. Gather together the highest fiber (low carbohydrate) foods you can eat. This list includes: onions, zucchini, rutabagas, bok choy, Chinese cabbage, turnips, garlic, cabbage, dinosaur kale, broccoli, carrots, celery, and cauliflower. Include raw seeds of: sesame, sunflower and pumpkin. Include grains & legumes of millet, quinoa, amaranth, lentils, barley and oats (steel cut or rolled). *Exclude wheat, rice, corn, and soy.* Get 3-5 large cans of Natural Goodness Chicken broth, or make your own vegetable broth. You can also use as a soup base Knudsen's brand "Very Veggie" - which is similar to V8 juice, but all organic. **As you are cleansing, it is even more imperative than ever to use ALL organic ingredients!**

During your program, make your meals out of these substances. That means you can stir-sauté (*instead of stir frying in oil*) the cooked grains and veggies in a wok. You can make soup out of these vegetables, grains and seeds. Use your imagination! Eat as much of the soup with the low carbohydrate veggies as possible. After you have cooked the soup, and it is in your bowl, add the PLC's of your choice, according to your taste buds. Use turmeric, cinnamon, onion, garlic and ginger. For your emotional balance during this time use Rainmaker in your water, and alternate with Green Dragon. Drink at least one quart of water per 50 pounds of weight on your body.

ForeverGreen makes a protein supplement called Thunder, which contains probiotics (friendly intestinal bacteria) and enzymes, vitamins and minerals. This is good to have once or twice a day, along with the above-mentioned substances. In rebuilding our GI tract, it is important to re-establish the proper quantity of friendly intestinal bacteria, which enhances our immune system. Most of us are deficient in enzymes, therefore we should build up our supply.

Gall Bladder Refresher

Get two gallons of organic apple juice or cider. If you have a juicer, you may make the apple juice fresh, which will provide a higher vitality drink. Drink one gallon of this juice each day. If hungry, you may eat apples.

I suggest the addition of a few drops cinnamon to one glass of juice. Have the next glass plain apple juice. The next glass, add a couple drops of ginger. While frankincense & nutmeg are of useful support for the gall bladder, some may not want to add them to the juice. In this case, take a teaspoon before bedtime.

During the day, it is also a good practice to use Rainmaker once or twice in a full glass of alkaline water.

The evening after your second day of drinking the apple juice mixture, combine 1/2 cup organic, virgin olive oil with the juice of one lemon and 1/4 teaspoon lemongrass PLC. Drink this down. I usually have a dry cracker handy after I've ingested the olive oil mixture, and chew this up afterwards. This takes the oily residues out of my mouth. In the morning after this cleanse, you may have a bowel movement which is either very green, or there could be green pellets in the toilet bowl. These are the gall stones you have expelled. *There is a combination Liver and Gall Bladder refresher listed under Liver.*

Immune System Enhancement

Many of the aqueous Plant Life Concentrates in this booklet are antibacterial, antifungal and antiviral. Some say they are an immunostimulant, antimicrobial, or anti-infectious. This means that when you use any of the PLC's with these health properties, no matter if you are doing a liver cleanse or taking a bath with one of the combinations, you are going to be positively impacting your immune system.

Rev. Hanna Kroeger gave us a powerful procedure to enhance our immune system, though it was messy. We would finely mince onions and mash cloves of garlic. Then, we put these along the spine and cover with a hot towel. She taught that this was a good way to pull virus out of the spine, and allow the properties of onion and garlic to be pulled along the nerves (*which exit between the vertebrae*) to the various organs which they supply.

She said this was also useful in cases of meningitis (where one or more of the 3 protective coverings around the brain get infected or inflamed.) In that case it is important to put the onion and garlic high up on the neck, and into the back of the scalp.

Now we have a much more simple way to do this with the onion and garlic PLC's. Just drizzle them along either side of the spine, massage in, cover with a warm towel, and then cover with a dry towel.

Eliminating Inflammatory
Processes in The Body

Why do we have so much inflammation? Inflammation is the local tissue response to injury. The injury may come from a traumatic blow, introduction of a foreign body, chemicals, microorganisms, worms and parasites, electrical and radiation damage. One of the greatest causes of tissue damage is a chronic level of acidosis (*too much acid*) in the body.

The way we describe where the inflammation takes place is through medical terminology, and the last 4 letters in the word are "itis". If a nerve is inflamed, we call it neuritis. If the liver is inflamed, we call it hepatitis. When there is inflammation, there is usually pain as well.

When injury occurs, histamine is released, the body increases heat, and blood vessels dilate to increase circulation to the damaged tissue. White blood cells enter in to help "eat up" the damaged particles. The lymphatic system comes in to help carry away the excess fluid. If the inflammation happens in a short amount of time, it is termed acute. If the inflammation is of a longstanding time period, it is termed chronic. It is the chronic inflammation we are most concerned about. This means there is some agent, which the body is holding onto, which continues to keep the tissues irritated and hot.

One cause of chronic inflammation is a liver that is congested and can't do its job. If so, you may want to go on a Liver Cleanse (*mentioned in this section.*) Inflammation can also come from allergies, which usually stem from a congested liver. If parasites are causing inflammation, do a worm and parasite cleanse.

When one has an easily reached more external inflammatory process, where it resides in joints, muscles, or over a particular area (such as the throat, chest, intestines, etc.) use the ginger or rosemary compress, as described earlier, over the affected area.

In addition, make it a regular practice for at least 30 days of including as many of the PLC's in this list as you can handle: astaxanthin, basil, Green Dragon, chili, frankincense, nutmeg, ginger, onion, peppermint, sage, turmeric, cinnamon and White Dragon. Remember to begin slowly, and then gradually add more PLC's when you can handle them. If you overload the system with too much, too quickly, you may make the condition worse, before it gets better.

Use these PLC's in your drinking water, in juices; rub them on your body over the affected areas. Some of the PLC's will taste better in fruit juices, and others will taste better in vegetable juices. Experiment and see what works for you. Generally 1/4 teaspoon total of the PLC's is sufficient in one pint (16 oz.) of juice or water. You can mix them in any amount you choose.

If you feel your inflammation is due to excessive acid levels (low pH) in the body, one must eliminate certain low pH beverages (coffee, caffeinated tea, soda, alcohol), and go on a specialized diet, which we will not describe in this booklet.[15]

For general purposes in healing inflammation (not focusing on the pH factor), choose a very simple diet. If you are used to eating a lot of animal proteins, you may choose to go on a vegetarian diet, or substitute animal proteins with fish. If you are a vegetarian, you may choose to simplify your diet to just the basics. Eliminate dairy products. In general, the more simple the diet, the better, as the body will have a greater chance of focusing on clearing the inflammation. Don't use any polyunsaturated oils. Use coconut oil, raw cultured butter from grass-fed cows, or no fats at all.

[15] Please refer to Dr. Mark Cochran's book on balancing pH and alkalizing the body.

Kidneys & Urinary System

The kidneys do an amazing job of filtering our blood, 24 hours a day. The kidneys have an important job of regulating mineral levels in the body. They retain the minerals we need, and excrete the rest. However, if our kidneys are damaged, they may let go of too many minerals. This can cause nutritional deficiencies and make our body too acidic. The kidneys produce urine to keep our internal fluids at the appropriate level. When we are dehydrated, it causes a greater burden on our kidneys. The combination of an acid condition plus not drinking enough fluids can predispose one to kidney stones.

One of the most supportive practices to help our kidneys is to drink our required amount of water daily. This is either one-quart per 50 pounds of body weight, or take your body weight and divide that in half. This will give you the number of ounces of pure water to drink. You can add any of the following Plant Life concentrates, to your drinking water, which are supportive to the kidneys and urinary system - cardamom, chamomile, cinnamon, frankincense, geranium, lemon, orange and parsley.

One to Three-Day Refresher
for Kidneys & Liver

You may also choose to go on a one to three day refresher for the kidneys and entire urinary system. These same practices also support the liver. There are many ways you can refresh the kidneys and liver. Here are some suggestions. Mix and match these ideas with what appeals to you.

1. To one gallon of water, add one tablespoon of the Green Dragon. Other additions to this water can be freshly juiced lemons, limes, chili and lemongrass. A natural sweetener may be added, if desired such as Yacon.

2. Eat an entirely alkaline diet of raw vegetables. Cut up vegetables and munch throughout the day. Don't use any fatty dips or dressings. Drink water as listed in #1 above.

3. Instead of eating the raw veggies, you may choose to juice them. The kidneys and liver both love raw greens - celery, kale, cabbage, collard greens, cucumber, carrot and beet. PLC's can be added to these fresh vegetable juices, according to your taste. This is a good opportunity to see which PLC's you enjoy most!

4. One might also add lightly steamed greens (kale, collard greens, spinach) and organic asparagus. Be sure to drink the cooking water from asparagus. The aqueous Plant Life Concentrates of lemongrass, garlic, ginger and onion are tasty additions to your vegetables.

5. Both the kidneys and liver enjoy beets and freshly juiced lemons. The beets can either be cooked or juiced raw.

6. When watermelon is in season, get an organic watermelon and juice the entire fruit - rind and all. Or, just juice the red part. This cleanses the bloodstream as well as gives the kidneys an opportunity to "clean house." One can add the Red Dragon to watermelon juice for a wonderful flavor sensation and nutrient support.

Liver Refresher

For 2-3 days, eat all the tomatoes and drink all the tomato juice you can. I like to make a soup from tomato juice, diced stewed tomatoes, with chopped onions, some chopped parsley (or other greens) and green peppers. Then when this mixture is in your soup bowl, add the PLC's of onion, garlic, chili, turmeric, ginger, lemongrass, basil, rosemary, sage and thyme. You may alternate by using 1-3 of these PLC's in different bowls of your soup. You don't have to have them all in one bowl, which could be overwhelming. I like to alternate glasses of fresh lemon juice (1-2 tablespoons of the juice to a 10-12 ounce glass of water with Yacon) one hour, and then have a glass of tomato juice another hour. I like to add 1-2 the PLC's mentioned above to my tomato juice.

On the night when you have completed your lemon and tomato cleansing, mix together the following "cocktail":

3-4 ounces (1/3 to 1/2 cup) olive oil

2 ounces (1/4 cup) castor oil

The juice of 3 oranges and 2 lemons

A little water can be added, if desired.

Drink this down, and go immediately to bed, lying on your right side. In the middle of the night or the next morning, you will feel the urge to dash to the toilet. You will be excreting all the black, stagnant bile your gall bladder has been holding. It will usually have the smell of turpentine. I suggest doing this re-fresher cleanse so that the day after you drink the "cocktail", you don't have to go to work. Some people may feel nauseated for a little while in the morning, or may need to make several trips to the toilet to expel the waste. However, after you are complete with all you will expel, you will find an amazing sense of light-ness and mental clarity you haven't felt in a long time. You may also notice your attitude has improved. If you were depressed, lethargic or just bogged down mentally, you will notice either this is completely gone, or greatly diminished.

Alternative Refresher: Some people may not be able to tolerate tomatoes. If so, then substitute freshly juiced carrots, and fast on this juice for one to two days. The same PLC's can be mixed into your carrot juice. I especially love the Red Dragon mixed in my carrot juice. At another time, you can mix the Green Dragon into your juice. After you have completed your cleanse, have the same "cocktail" mentioned above.

Combination Liver & Gall Bladder Refresher

Get a one-gallon glass jar. Juice two small beets and beet greens. Add this to the jar. Add one cup fresh lemon juice and 2-4 tablespoons natural sweetener, such as Yacon. Add one half-gallon (2 quarts) of water. You may now add any of the PLC's that you desire. Good choices include chili, ginger and the Green Dragon. Please drink an additional two quarts of plain high alkaline (pH 8-9) water.

You don't need to ingest the oil "cocktail" mentioned in the previous refreshers. If this is your first time cleansing your liver and gall bladder, I recommend this particular refresher. Remember the emotional component mentioned at the beginning of this section regarding these refreshers. When doing the liver, gall bladder cleanses, the emotions come into play more often than with the other refreshers. The Rainmaker may be useful to sip on throughout your refreshing cleanse.

The Whole Body Cleanse

Any time we abstain from eating our usual diet, and focus on liquids, mixed with PLC's, we will give our entire body a chance to relax, detoxify and rebuild. We could call this a master cleanse because it will help all parts of the body. It will help you expel excess mucus, will reduce inflammation and will add volume to your blood so that it can be filtered by the kidneys and excreted in the urine. It will add moisture to your intestines, which could cause extra bowel movements. If you have some diarrhea or loose stools, just bless them and be OK with this.

I suggest going on this cleanse on a weekend, or when you have a couple days when you don't have your usual work responsibilities. Some people will book a room at a hot springs hotel, and use this as a mini-vacation. This is really the very best, as it is the most loving to your body when you don't have other demands upon your mind, emotions or your body. *It can also be an opportune time for a spiritual reconnection.*

Let someone else have the pleasure of caring for your children or spouse for a couple of days! When you return, you will be much more available for your family and your work activities. If you choose to go to a hot springs, the hot mineral water heated from the Earth will help the pores of your skin (*the largest organ in your body*) open up. You will take in minerals you need, and expel toxins. How lovely!

This is the basic format of this cleanse, which you can do for one or two days, and up to 28 days if you are accustomed to fasting. Drink at least a gallon of water a day. Note that for a **Maintenance Dosage**, you drink one half your body weight in water. However, for a **Therapeutic (Detoxification) Dosage**, you drink one ounce of water per pound of weight on your body. There are 128 ounces in a gallon of water. This means that if you weigh 128 pounds, you would ingest a gallon of fluid daily, for as many days as you choose to fast. Those that weigh more would drink more fluids accordingly.

What to mix in your water? The traditional whole body re-fresher usually uses the fresh juices of lemon, lime, chili and some kind of sweetener (*Yacon or Yakave*). This is the base. Then, you may add any of the other PLC's as you desire. I suggest that you mix up into a one-gallon container the basic recipe. Then, as you pour out a glass, you may wish to add a few drops of the PLC's of your choice. This is a wonderful way to experiment with the PLC's to see what they will do for your body constitution and chemistry.

If you have had a history of constipation or do not have 2-3 bowel movements each day, you may choose to have a series of colonic irrigations during your cleanse. This is optional. If you go on this cleanse for more than 2-3 days, you may find that you naturally will begin to expel a lot of old fecal matter. Each of us is different, and it is important to honor your body constitution and rhythms.

Removing Worms and Parasites

Worms and parasites are present in our body when we have a weak immune system, when our system is acidic and when our body has many poisons. Some of these poisons/toxins include heavy metals, genetically modified substances, chemicals, pesticides and environmental toxins. One of the most damaging aspects of having worms and parasites in our bodies is the waste, which these "critters" excrete. This can worsen an already acidic pH, can lead to anxiety, depression, inflammation, irritation, apathy, listlessness, brain fog, and much more.

Those who are a host to worms and parasites in their bodies often exhibit a kind of "nervous energy". They will bounce or shake their legs up and down while the toes are on the floor. They may drum their fingers across a desktop. They may be unable to sleep at night, or grind their teeth at night. In chil-dren, often pinworms cause a child to itch the anus in their sleep. And then, as children will often suck on their thumb or fingers, they re-introduce the eggs into the body. Some causes of ADD or ADHD are worm and parasite infestation.

The following aqueous PLC's that are described in this book are useful in removing worms and parasites: cardamom, chamomile, clove, lemon, neroli, nutmeg, peppermint, rosemary, spearmint and ginger. In order to obtain all of these PLC's, it is necessary to use Rainmaker, Green, Red and White Dragons in addition to rosemary.

With many of the other cleanses, you will also be gradually addressing the removal of worms and parasites. However, if you feel that worms and parasites are your major health concern, you may desire to go on a refreshing cleanse just for this purpose. If so, mix one teaspoon each of the white, green and Red Dragons, plus 1/2 teaspoon rosemary in at least one gallon of pure high pH water (8-9 pH). You may go on this cleanse for 1-3 days. If you go on the cleanse longer than one day, you may choose to mix your PLC's in tomato juice one day, and grape, carrot or apple juice another day.

Substances, which worms and parasites do not like, include onion, garlic, ginger root, pumpkin seeds and calimyrna figs. While drinking your chosen liquid mixed with these aqueous Plant Life Concentrates, you may enjoy a high fiber diet. Use your intuition and your imagination. Eat a bowl of whole grain rice (there are many varieties other than just brown rice). Add some of the PLC's to your rice. Have a bowl of rolled-grain cereal. Use a combination of oats, rye, barley, etc. I suggest refraining from using wheat for this experience. Cook the rolled grains in apple juice and water. When the cooking is finished, top your cereal with raw pumpkin seeds, figs, sunflower seeds, flax seeds, sesame seeds, rice or almond milk and White Dragon.

There are two types of fibers - soluble and insoluble. Soluble fiber (oat bran, apple pectin, etc.) works on the internal organs, and if used in this cleansing diet, will help to expel worms and parasites in these places. Insoluble fiber helps scrub the intestines clean.

Many times, worm and parasite supplements taken in capsule form only work on worms and parasites in the intestinal tract. The reason this does not solve the problem is that there are worms and parasites in the brain, in the heart (especially prominent around the heart valves), in the liver, in the lungs, and other organs. When we only cleanse the intestines, these other worms and parasites lay their eggs, and the new "critters" then move into the intestines.

When we ingest soluble fibers, and mix these with *anthelminthic* aqueous PLC's, we get the worms out of these other places. In order to get the worms and parasites out of the brain, I suggest adding frankincense and nutmeg along with other PLC's in this list. That way, the frankincense will bond with and carry these other substances in the brain.

Glossary

Anti-inflammatory—a substance that counteracts inflammation

Anthelminthic—a substance which removes worms and parasites

Antimicrobial—a substance that prevents harmful effects in the human body from microbes (bacteria, fungus, virus, etc.)

Antioxidant—counteracts the effects of free radicals

Antiseptic—preventing decay in tissue and also the spread of microorganisms throughout the body

Antispasmodic—preventing or relieving spasms

Astringent—a classification within the herbal kingdom - that which draws together; tightens tissues which have loosened and become flaccid

Bile—contains bile salts, cholesterol, bile pigments, lecithin, lipids and electrolytes; produced in the liver and secreted into the duodenum and also gall bladder for additional storage - for the purpose of digesting fats

Blood Brain Barrier—three protective membranes surrounding the brain (dura, arachnoid and pia mater) which help prevent toxins from entering the brain

Candida albicans—a yeast-like fungus, a normal part of our intestinal system; it easily gets out of balance and grows in disproportionate amounts when certain friendly bacteria are killed off by the use of antibiotics. When it invades other areas of the body (in a systemic manner) there are many unpleasant symptoms.

Candidiasis—the condition of having an over population of the Candida albicans organisms

Carminative—a substance that promotes the elimination of intestinal gas

Cholesterol—a sterol (alcohol) occurring in animal foods, and also produced in the liver; a constituent in bile and a precursor to steroid (sex) hormones.

Degenerative Conditions—That which affects several systems, and is a chronic, slowly evolving condition. Examples include allergies, arthritis, asthma, diabetes, hypertension, insomnia and neurological conditions..

Endothelium—a type of flat cell which lines blood and lymphatic vessels

Flatulence—intestinal gas

HDL—high-density lipids; the kind that are favorable to our health

Homocysteine—when not converted to cystathione, and in the absence of adequate vitamin B6, homocysteine is a free radical that attacks the arteries

Immunostimulant—a substance which has a positive impact upon the immune system

"itis" conditions—I use this term when referring to places where inflammation causes pain, loss of oxygen in the body. Some examples are arthritis, bronchitis, hepatitis, and conjunctivitis. Any word, which ends with "itis", can generally be helped with substances that exhibit anti-inflammatory properties.

Jaundice—a condition in which the skin and "whites of the eyes" have a yellowish pigment; comes from excessive bile in system due to blockage of bile, or other problems in the body; important to have checked out as to cause

Law of Signature—a way of observing certain characteristics of plants which allows us to know what area of the human body it works with

LDL—low-density lipids; the kind that are unfavorable to our health

Liver Enzyme Systems—superoxide dismutase (SOD) and glutathione peroxidase - two free radical control substances produced in the liver

Mucolytic—a substance which dissolves excess mucus in body

Platelets—substances in the blood which help when tissue is damaged. They come in to plug the "hole" left by trauma, and clot blood. When the body is in a continuous state of inflammation and acidosis, there can be too many platelets, which clump together, causing the blood to thicken and cause problems

Sedative—a substance that produces a soothing effect, calming hyperactive nerves and reducing anxiety; can help induce sleep.

Spasm—an involuntary contraction of muscle tissue, often involving pain. A strong spasm produces menstrual cramps, and in a severe form can cause epileptic seizures

Terrain Theory—rather than looking at disease as being caused by some outside agent, we look at the internal factors such as pH, level of free radicals (internal radiation), toxins present, etc.. When we change the internal terrain of the body, disease doesn't have a chance!

Tonic—an agent that produces or restores proper tone (strength)to the body

Xenobiotic—an artificial estrogen-like substance produced by exposure to environmental toxins; found in high amounts in those who are estrogen-dominant. We also increase xenobiotic substances by heating food in a plastic container in a microwave oven.

About Dr. Marcy Foley

Dr. Marcy Foley is an innovator in Natural Healing. Her Health Readings, books, teachings and healing sessions have helped people in over 15 countries to regain their health using only natural therapies.

Dr. Foley works very deeply with her well-being recipients. She attributes the success of her work because she integrates the physical, emotional, mental and spiritual areas of one's life. She recognizes the importance of tuning into one's thoughts, feelings and spiritual foundation for attainment of one's wellness goals. Dr. Foley believes that it is each person's free choice to find the Higher Power of their own understanding.

Biographical Information:

- B.S. in Natural Foods Nutrition, Donsbach University, 1980
- Doctor of Chiropractic, Palmer College of Chiropractic, 1985
- Certificate in Healing Ministry, Universal Life Church, 1986
- Physicians Training, National Center for Homeopathy, 1991
- Master Herbalist, The School of Natural Healing, 1993
- Doctor of Naturopathy, American Naturopathic Medical Association, 1993

Dr. Foley's Publications

- *Psychometric Aura Reading*, 1990
- *Integrating Your Wholeness: A Reference Guide To Assist You in Merging With Your Internal Physician* (reprinted 13 times, last printing 1999)
- *Akanthos: A Book of Spiritual Insights*; Foley and Young, 1991
- *The Alchemist's Handbook to Homeopathy*; Hardy, Nonman, Foley, 1994
- *Embraced By the Essence: Your Journey into Wellness Using Pure Quality Essential Oils*, 1998, 2000
- *Illuminating Physical Experience*; Foley, Shaffer, Davidsson, 2000

Contacting Dr. Marcy Foley

Marcy Foley is not a medical physician. Therefore, she cannot give advice on diagnosed conditions or recommend remedies or practices for disease conditions. Dr. Foley works from the standpoint of prevention, cleansing and rebuilding the body so it is able to function optimally. If you would like assistance from Dr. Foley in creating a personalized natural care wellness program, please send inquiries to:

P.O. Box 783, Lyons, CO   80503
drmarcy@kornax.com

Dr. Foley is not at this time available by telephone. Please be patient. Dr. Foley does answer all inquires, however at times the demand from well-being recipients is extensive. She answers requests in the order in which she receives them.

Appendix A—Map of Taste Receptors Diagram.

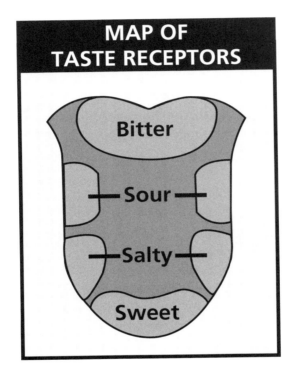

Appendix B—Free Radicals Diagram.

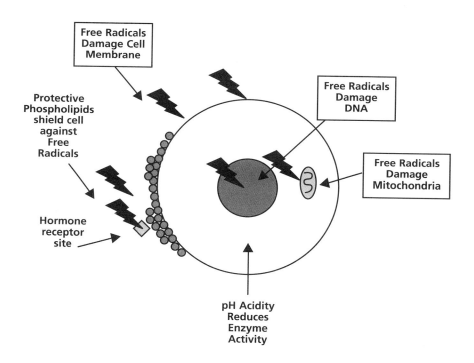

Free Radicals
Damage Cell
Membrane

Free Radicals
Damage
DNA

Protective
Phospholipids
shield cell
against
Free
Radicals

Free Radicals
Damage
Mitochondria

Hormone
receptor
site

pH Acidity
Reduces
Enzyme
Activity